Beyond Weight Loss for Women

The Role and Effects of Hormones in Weight Loss.

ANN R. MOSIER

1

COPYRIGHT ©

ABOUT THE AUTHOR

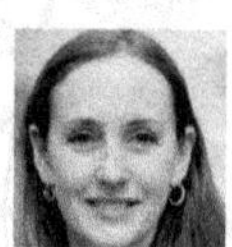

Ann R. Mosier is a passionate advocate for women's health and wellness, with a particular focus on postpartum care and weight management. As a mother herself, she understands the unique challenges and triumphs of the postpartum journey and is dedicated to empowering women to prioritize their physical and emotional well-being after childbirth. With a background in Exercise Therapy, Mosier brings a wealth of knowledge and expertise to her writing, offering practical advice, evidence-based strategies, and heartfelt encouragement to women navigating the complexities of postpartum weight loss. Through her compassionate and relatable approach, she strives to inspire and support women as they reclaim their health, confidence, and vitality after giving birth. Mosier is committed to promoting a holistic approach to postpartum wellness, recognizing the interconnectedness of physical, emotional, and mental well-being. She believes in the power of self-care, self-compassion, and self-love as essential components of the postpartum journey, and she is dedicated to helping women cultivate a positive and empowering relationship with their bodies and themselves. In addition to her writing, Mosier is a certified Women Health Coach. She is deeply passionate about sharing her knowledge and experience with others, and she is honored to be a part of each woman's journey towards health, happiness, and self-discovery.

When she's not writing or working with clients, Mosier enjoys spending time with her family, practicing yoga, and exploring nature. She resides in Los Angeles with her husband and children where she finds inspiration and joy in the everyday moments of motherhood. Through her work, Mosier hopes to empower women to embrace their postpartum journey with confidence, resilience, and grace, knowing that they are capable of achieving their goals and living their best lives, both for themselves and for their families.

DISCLAIMER

The information provided in this book is for educational and informational purposes only. It is not intended as a substitute for professional medical advice, diagnosis, or treatment. Always seek the advice of your physician or other qualified healthcare provider with any questions you may have regarding a medical condition or the suitability of any recommendations provided in this book.

The author and publisher of this book make no representations or warranties regarding the accuracy, completeness, or efficacy of the information contained herein. The author and publisher disclaim any liability for any loss or damage incurred by readers or users of this book, directly or indirectly, as a result of the information provided or any actions taken based on the content of this book.

Individual results may vary. The effectiveness of any recommendations or strategies discussed in this book depends on various factors, including but not limited to an individual's health status, medical history, genetics, lifestyle, and adherence to the recommendations provided. Readers are encouraged to consult with healthcare professionals before implementing any changes to their diet, exercise routine, or medical treatment plan.

The inclusion of product names, brands, or specific treatment modalities in this book does not constitute an endorsement or recommendation by the author or publisher. Readers are advised to conduct their own research and exercise discretion when considering any products, services, or treatments mentioned in this book.

By reading this book, you acknowledge and agree to the terms of this disclaimer. If you do not agree with these terms, you should not use or rely on the information provided in this book.

11

CHAPTER 1~ *INTRODUCTION*

UNDERSTANDING THE COMPLEXITIES OF WEIGHT LOSS

Our brains drive us to eat for a variety of reasons; occasionally, they are motivated by true hunger, and other times they are emotional in nature. The issue arises when a person's brain consistently signals them to eat even when they're not hungry. Regular overeating and different eating disorders may result from this.

An equation is typically used to describe weight management: energy in, or the calories we consume through food and drink, must equal energy out, or the calories we expend, in order to prevent weight gain or reduction. We will lose weight if we expend more calories than we consume, and vice versa.

Many people believe that losing weight is as simple as ingesting less calories than one burns. Although this idea is fundamentally correct, the reality is much more complex, particularly for women. The hormonal environment of the female body adds a level of complexity that has a big impact on weight control.

Hormonal Effects

Hormones are essential for controlling a number of physiological functions, such as hunger and metabolism. Hormone fluctuations during the menstrual cycle, pregnancy, perimenopause, and menopause can have a significant effect on how women regulate their weight. It is essential to comprehend the interactions between hormones including estrogen, progesterone, insulin, cortisol, and thyroid hormones when creating weight loss plans that work for women's specific needs.

Variability in Metabolism

Women have a variety of metabolic profiles that are influenced by age, genetics, body type, and way of life. Individual differences can be noted in metabolic rate, nutrition consumption efficiency, and fat distribution patterns. Appreciating and honoring these metabolic variations is crucial to creating customized weight reduction programs that last.

Psychological Elements

In addition to physiological variables, psychological factors have a significant impact on the results of weight loss. Even the most carefully planned diets and fitness regimens can be derailed by emotional eating, stress, negative body image, and social pressures. It is essential to address the psychological components of weight control in order to promote resilience, a positive outlook, and long-term commitment to healthy practices.

Environmental Elements

There are many obesogenic cues in the modern world that encourage overeating and sedentary behavior. Obesity is becoming more common due to easy access to high-calorie foods, widespread marketing of harmful items, and sedentary lifestyles. Fighting the obesity pandemic requires developing conditions that are conducive of stress management, physical activity, and a nutritious diet.

Understanding that losing weight involves a complex interaction of hormonal, metabolic, psychological, and environmental components rather than just counting calories in and out emphasizes the value of taking a holistic approach. Through a complete approach to weight loss, women can attain long-lasting outcomes, improve their general well-being, and maximize their health.

IMPORTANCE OF HORMONAL BALANCE IN WOMEN'S HEALTH

Maintaining hormonal equilibrium is essential to the healthy operation of every system in the female body. A woman's hormones might become "out of whack," which can lead to a number of undesirable outcomes.

Every woman will go through typical, transient symptoms related to hormone balance. Hormones are chemicals that communicate with your organs, skin, muscles, and other tissues through your bloodstream to regulate various bodily activities. Your body receives these messages and knows what to do and when. Your health and life depend on hormones.

The following are some reasons why hormonal balance is important:1. Regulates Metabolism: Metabolism, which includes the creation, storage, and use of energy, depends on hormonal balance. Insulin, thyroid hormones, and leptin are examples of hormones that are essential for controlling metabolism, making sure that nutrients are used effectively, and avoiding weight gain or loss.

2. Promotes Reproductive Health: Women's reproductive health depends on hormonal balance. Ovulation, fertility, and the menstrual cycle are all regulated by hormones like progesterone and estrogen. Reproductive diseases such as infertility and irregular menstruation can be caused by imbalances in these hormones.

3. Affects Mood and Mental Health: Hormones affect mood, emotional stability, and cognitive function by influencing neurotransmitter activity in the brain. Mood disorders including melancholy, anxiety, and irritability can be exacerbated by hormonal imbalances in the body, including those involving serotonin, dopamine, cortisol, and estrogen.

4. Preserves Bone Health: Hormonal equilibrium is necessary to preserve bone strength and density. Because it promotes bone growth and prevents bone resorption, estrogen is essential for bone metabolism. Estrogen imbalances can raise the risk

of osteoporosis and bone fractures, especially following menopause.

5. Controls Stress Response: The body's reaction to stress is regulated by hormone balance. The adrenal glands create hormones like cortisol, which assist the body deal with stress by promoting energy reserves and reducing inflammation. Hormonal equilibrium can be upset by prolonged stress, which can have a negative impact on health.

6. Regulates Hunger and Weight: Hormones are important for controlling hunger, fullness, and body weight. Hormones including insulin, ghrelin, and leptin send signals to the brain about hunger and fullness, which affects how much food is consumed and how much energy is used. These hormone imbalances have been linked to obesity, weight gain, and overeating.

7. Promotes Skin Health: Keeping your hormones in check is essential to having healthy skin. Estrogen and testosterone are two examples of hormones that affect the formation of collagen, moisture, and oil in the skin. Hormonal imbalances may be a factor in skin disorders such acne, dermatitis, and early aging.

When you have excessive amounts of one or more hormones, you have an imbalance in your hormone levels. It's an umbrella term that can include a broad spectrum of illnesses related to hormones.

Hormones are potent messengers.
Even though you may have somewhat too much or too little of a hormone, many hormones can have major effects on your body and lead to issues that

require treatment. The severity of hormonal imbalances can vary, ranging from short-term to long-term.

CONDITIONS CAUSED BY HORMONAL IMBALANCE

Hormone problems are the root cause of numerous medical disorders. For the majority of hormones, either too much or too little causes symptoms and health issues. While many of these imbalances require medical intervention, others of them are temporary and may go away on their own. Among the most prevalent disorders linked to hormones are:

An irregular menstrual cycle: The menstrual cycle is influenced by a number of hormones. As a result, an imbalance in any one or more of those hormones may induce irregular periods.
A few hormone-related disorders that can lead to irregular periods are amenorrhea and polycystic ovarian syndrome (PCOS).
Infertility: In individuals assigned female at birth, hormonal abnormalities are the main cause of infertility. Infertility can result from disorders connected to hormones, such as PCOS and anovulation. In addition to hormonal problems that impact fertility, people assigned to the masculine gender at birth may also have hypogonadism, or low testosterone.

Acne: Blocked pores are the main cause of acne. Hormonal variations, particularly throughout puberty, are a crucial component in the development of acne, although there are numerous other causes as well. Hormones that become active throughout puberty stimulate oil glands, including those in the skin of your face.

Adult acne, or hormonal acne: Hormonal fluctuations cause your skin to generate more oil, which leads to the development of hormonal acne. This is most prevalent in those going through menopause, pregnant women, and those on testosterone medication.

Diabetes: The most prevalent endocrine (hormone-related) illness in the US is diabetes. Diabetes is characterized by insufficient or absent pancreatic production of the hormone insulin or by improper body utilization of it. Diabetes comes in a variety of forms. Type 2 diabetes, Type 1 diabetes, and gestational diabetes are the most prevalent types. Diabetes needs to be managed.

Thyroid disease: Hypothyroidism (low thyroid hormone levels) and hyperthyroidism (high thyroid hormone levels) are the two main forms of thyroid disease. Every ailment has a variety of potential causes. Treatment is necessary for thyroid disease.

Obesity: An imbalance in some hormones can lead to weight increase in the form of stored fat since many hormones can influence how your body uses energy and signals when you need food. For instance, low thyroid hormones (hypothyroidism) and high levels of the hormone cortisol can both lead to obesity.

Unbalanced hormone levels can lead to weight gain and include:

Hypothyroidism: This disorder is characterized by low thyroid hormone levels, which slow down your metabolism. Gaining weight could result from this.

A rare disorder known as Cushing's syndrome is brought on by an excess of the hormone cortisol in the body. Rapid weight gain occurs in the chest, back of your neck (sometimes referred to as "buffalo hump"), abdomen, and face (also referred to as "moon face").

Menopause: Because of hormonal changes that slow down their metabolism, many women gain weight during menopause. Remembering that this type of "hormonal imbalance" is typical and expected in life is crucial.

In general, hormonal balance affects several physiological processes, including metabolism, reproduction, mood, and skin health, making it crucial for general health and wellbeing. For optimum health, it is essential to maintain hormonal balance through stress reduction techniques, a balanced lifestyle, and medical interventions as needed..

CHAPTER 2 ~ FOUNDATIONS OF HORMONAL REGULATION

OVERVIEW OF HORMONES INVOLVED IN WEIGHT LOSS

Our hunger, metabolism, and distribution of body fat are influenced by the hormones leptin, insulin, sex hormones, and growth hormones. These hormones are more prevalent in overweight people, which promotes an irregular metabolism and the buildup of body fat.

The endocrine system is a network of glands that secretes hormones into our blood. In order to help our body deal with various situations and challenges, the endocrine system collaborates with the immune system and the nervous system. Hormone excesses or deficiencies can cause weight gain, but weight gain itself can cause hormonal alterations.

The connection between being overweight and leptin

Fat cells create the hormone leptin, which is then released into the bloodstream. By influencing particular brain regions, leptin lowers an individual's appetite and lessens their desire to eat. It appears to regulate the body's storage of body fat as well.

Since fat is the source of leptin, individuals who are overweight typically have higher levels of leptin than those who are normal weight. But even though overweight persons have higher levels of this hormone that suppresses hunger, they are less sensitive to the effects of leptin and hence don't always feel full during and after meals. The question of why fat people's brains aren't receiving leptin signals is still being investigated.

The Connection Between Insulin and Being Overweight

The pancreas secretes the hormone insulin, which is critical for controlling how fat and carbs are metabolized. Insulin promotes the uptake of glucose, or sugar, from the blood into tissues like fat, muscles, and liver. This procedure is crucial for maintaining appropriate blood glucose levels and ensuring that energy is accessible for daily activities.

Sometimes insulin signals are lost in an overweight individual, and their tissues lose their ability to regulate glucose levels. Metabolic syndrome and type II diabetes may result from this.

Relationship Between Overweight and Sex Hormones

The distribution of body fat is a significant factor in the development of diseases linked to obesity, including heart disease, stroke, and several types of arthritis. Compared to fat accumulated on our thighs, hips, and bottom, fat surrounding our abdomen increases our risk of disease. It appears that the distribution of body fat is influenced by both androgens and oestrogens. Premenopausal women's ovaries produce oestrogens, which are sex hormones. They trigger the ovulation process each menstrual cycle.

The testes (testicles) and ovaries of males and postmenopausal women do not produce a significant amount of estrogen. Rather than in their ovaries, which are still producing a significant quantity of oestrogen, the majority of their oestrogen is created in their body fat. The testes produce a large amount of androgens in younger males. These levels progressively drop as a man ages.

Changes in body fat distribution are linked to changes in men's and women's sex hormone levels as they age. Older men and women who have gone through menopause tend to store more fat around their abdomens ('apple-shaped'), whereas women of reproductive age tend to store fat in their lower bodies ('pear-shaped'). Women who are postmenopausal and taking oestrogen pills do not gain belly fat. Studies on animals have also demonstrated that insufficient oestrogen causes excessive weight gain.

Growth Hormone and Overweight: A Correlation

Growth hormone is a hormone that the brain's pituitary gland secretes and affects height as well as the development of bone and muscle. Metabolism is also impacted by growth hormone. Growth hormone levels have been observed to be lower in overweight individuals than in normal weight individuals.

The Association Between Inflammatory Elements and Obesity

Additionally, low-grade chronic inflammation within the adipose tissue is linked to being overweight. Overconsumption of fat stores triggers stress responses in fat cells, which in turn cause the cells to release pro-inflammatory substances and immune cells from the adipose (fat) tissue.

Obesity is linked to a lower quality of life and a shortened life span, as well as an increased risk of various diseases, such as stroke, cardiovascular disease, and multiple cancers. The source of oestrogen production is essential, as evidenced by the correlation between an increased risk of breast cancer and the higher production of oestrogens in the fat of older obese women.

Hormone levels in obese or overweight individuals promote the buildup of body fat. Overeating and irregular exercise appear to'reset' the body's appetite and fat distribution systems over time, increasing a person's physiological propensity to gain weight. The body resists any temporary disturbances, like crash diets, because it is constantly working to preserve equilibrium.

Numerous studies have demonstrated that following a low-kilojoule diet, a person's blood leptin level decreases. A person's hunger may increase and metabolism may slow down if their leptin levels are lower. This could provide some insight into why crash dieters typically put the weight back on. Leptin therapy may eventually assist dieters in long-term weight maintenance, but further research is required before this is practical.

Evidence suggests that the body can be retrained to lose extra body fat and keep it off with long-term behavioral adjustments like regular exercise and healthy nutrition. Additionally, research has demonstrated that reducing weight with bariatric surgery, a nutritious diet, and exercise improves insulin resistance, reduces inflammation, and helps regulate obesity hormones. Losing weight is also linked to a lower risk of heart disease, stroke, type II diabetes, and certain types of cancer.

FACTORS INFLUENCING HORMONAL IMBALANCE

Hormonal imbalance in women can be caused by a number of circumstances, some of which are as follows:

1. Stress: Prolonged stress can upset the delicate hormonal balance, especially cortisol, which the adrenal glands release in response to stress. Inconsistencies in other hormones, including progesterone, estrogen, and thyroid hormones, can result from high cortisol levels.

2. Diet and Nutrition: Hormonal imbalances can be caused by eating a poor diet high in processed foods, sweets, and harmful fats. Hormonal function can also be disrupted by nutrient shortages, especially in important vitamins and minerals like zinc, magnesium, and vitamin D.

3. Lifestyle Practices: Hormonal balance can be impacted by a sedentary lifestyle, a lack of exercise, and inconsistent sleep patterns. While insufficient sleep can interfere with circadian rhythms and hormone production, physical activity decreases stress, enhances insulin sensitivity, and helps regulate hormone levels.

4. Environmental Toxins: Hormone signaling and metabolism can be disrupted by exposure to environmental toxins, such as endocrine-disrupting chemicals (EDCs), which are present in plastics,

cosmetics, pesticides, and home goods. EDCs cause hormone imbalances and negative health effects by mimicking or blocking the function of hormones.

5. Medications and Birth Control: Hormonal contraceptives, hormone replacement therapy (HRT), and medications for mental health issues or thyroid problems are just a few examples of the pharmaceuticals that might alter hormone levels and cause imbalances. It's crucial to talk about possible side effects with medical professionals prior to beginning or stopping any medicine.

6. Age and Life Stage: Hormonal changes occur naturally during several times of life, including adolescence, menstruation, pregnancy, the perimenopause, and menopause. Hormonal abnormalities brought on by these shifts may be transient or long-lasting, impacting mood, metabolism, reproduction, and general health.

7. Medical illnesses: Hormonal balance can be upset by underlying medical illnesses such insulin resistance, thyroid issues, adrenal disorders, and polycystic ovarian syndrome (PCOS). Managing symptoms and enhancing health results require

treating the underlying ailment and resolving hormone abnormalities.

8. Genetics and Family History: Certain hormonal abnormalities and imbalances can be inherited by an individual. Women who have a family history of diabetes, thyroid issues, or PCOS may be more susceptible to hormonal abnormalities.

Comprehending these variables and implementing dietary adjustments, lifestyle adjustments, stress reduction methods, and obtaining medical guidance as required can aid in reestablishing hormonal equilibrium and advancing general health and wellness. To address a hormonal imbalance comprehensively, it is critical to understand its source.

CHAPTER 3 ~ HORMONAL
IMBALANCE AND WEIGHT GAIN

IMPACT OF ESTROGEN LEVELS ON METABOLISM

Many times regarded as the main hormone involved in female sex, estrogen regulates metabolism in a variety of ways. It affects several physiological systems in the body, including reproductive activities, and has a significant effect on metabolism. Estrogen levels can impact metabolism in the following ways:

1. Energy Expenditure: By affecting metabolic rate, or the rate at which the body consumes calories while at rest, estrogen contributes to the regulation of energy expenditure. Increased metabolic rate is linked to higher amounts of estrogen, which encourages higher energy expenditure even during periods of inactivity. This may help keep you from gaining weight and help you maintain a healthy weight.

2. Fat Distribution: Subcutaneous adipose tissue, or fat beneath the skin, is preferred for fat deposition over visceral adipose tissue, or fat surrounding internal organs, due to estrogen's influence on patterns of fat distribution in the body. Visceral fat is linked to insulin resistance, inflammation, and metabolic diseases; subcutaneous fat is thought to be less metabolically active and to have fewer health hazards.

3. Insulin Sensitivity: Estrogen increases the body's sensitivity to insulin, which makes it possible for cells to absorb glucose from the bloodstream and use it as fuel. Improved glucose metabolism and a lower incidence of insulin resistance and type 2 diabetes are linked to higher levels of estrogen. Insulin secretion, nutritional balance, and survival are all regulated by estrogen effects in pancreatic islet β-cells. A low estrogen level increases metabolic dysfunction, which increases the risk of obesity, metabolic syndrome, and type 2 diabetes. Because estrogen affects insulin sensitivity, blood sugar levels are regulated and excessive glucose buildup in the bloodstream is avoided.

4. Appetite Regulation: Through regulating the action of hormones and neurotransmitters involved in hunger and satiety signals, estrogen affects appetite regulation. Increased sensitivity to the hormone leptin, which indicates fullness, and decreased sensitivity to the hormone ghrelin, which promotes appetite, are linked to higher estrogen levels. This can aid in controlling food intake and avoiding overindulging, which helps with weight management.

5. Thermogenesis: The body produces heat through the metabolism of skeletal muscle and brown adipose tissue (BAT), and this process is aided by estrogen. Thermogenesis is a process that increases body temperature and aids in energy expenditure, especially in response to cold exposure. Elevated amounts of estrogen could amplify thermogenic activity, augmenting the burning of calories and improving metabolic efficiency.

6. Maintenance of Muscle Mass: Lean muscle mass is maintained by estrogen, which supports good metabolic health in general. Skeletal muscle tissue has estrogen receptors, and muscle protein synthesis, repair, and regeneration are all influenced by

estrogen signaling. Sufficient amounts of estrogen promote the development and maintenance of muscle, which can increase metabolism and ward against age-related muscle loss (sarcopenia).

THYROID FUNCTION AND ITS ROLE IN WEIGHT REGULATION.

The thyroid gland is a major factor in controlling weight because it regulates metabolism and energy expenditure.
Thyroxine (T4) and triiodothyronine (T3), the two main hormones produced by the thyroid gland, control metabolism by affecting almost all of the body's cell activities. The basal metabolic rate (BMR), or the amount of energy used while at rest, is influenced by several hormones, which regulate how quickly the body uses oxygen and calories to produce energy. In addition, basal metabolic rate—which controls how effectively the body burns calories to support essential bodily activities like breathing, circulation, and temperature regulation—is directly impacted by thyroid hormones. Despite ingesting less calories,

hypothyroidism, or low thyroid hormone levels, can cause a drop in BMR, which can result in weight gain or trouble decreasing weight.

Thyroid hormones affect how fats are broken down and used as fuel. They also have an impact on lipid metabolism. The body may have trouble using fat that has been deposited as fuel in hypothyroidism, which can result in weight gain and fat buildup, especially around the abdomen.
The integrity and proper operation of muscles depend on thyroid hormones. Weakness in the muscles, exhaustion, and low levels of physical activity can all lead to weight gain or trouble shedding weight in a condition such as hypothyroidism. In contrast, hyperthyroidism (the overproduction of thyroid hormone) can result in inadvertent weight loss and muscular atrophy.

Finally, through their effects on metabolism and energy balance, thyroid hormones can indirectly affect how appetite is regulated and how the digestive system works. Hypothyroidism is linked to slower digestion and decreased appetite, both of which can lead to weight gain. On the other hand, despite consuming more calories, hyperthyroidism can cause weight loss via increasing hunger and intestinal motility.

Thyroid problems can impact the body's fluid balance, resulting in dehydration or water retention. Reduced thyroid activity in hypothyroidism may lead to bloating and fluid retention, which can momentarily raise body weight. On the other hand, increased perspiration and fluid loss due to hyperthyroidism might result in dehydration and weight loss.

The mechanism by which the body produces heat is called thermogenesis, and thyroid hormones have an impact on this process. A higher thyroid function promotes thermogenesis, which raises energy expenditure and aids in weight loss. On the other hand, a lower thyroid activity lowers thermogenesis, which lowers calorie expenditure and increases the risk of weight gain.

Overall, a woman's thyroid function affects a lot of bodily functions, including metabolism, energy expenditure, hunger control, and body composition—all of which are critical for controlling weight. Sustaining a healthy and optimal body weight requires maintaining thyroid function.

IMPACT OF CORTISOL AND STRESS ON HORMONAL BALANCE AND WEIGHT

The body releases 50–60% of cortisol within the first 30–40 minutes of awakening, with levels subsequently decreasing throughout the day. Cortisol release is often closely correlated with the circadian cycle of the body.
Your brain's hypothalamus and pituitary gland control the hormone's synthesis and release.
The adrenal glands release cortisol and adrenaline when there is heightened stress. The body gets ready for a potentially dangerous scenario by raising energy and heart rate in response to this.
Although this reaction is typical, prolonged increases in cortisol may have unfavorable side effects.
Cortisol levels rising slightly in reaction to stress is common and unlikely to have harmful adverse effects.

The hormone cortisol increases the body's metabolism of fat and carbohydrates, giving it a boost in energy. This process increases hunger in addition to being necessary for survival in certain settings. In addition, cravings for salty, fatty, and sweet meals might be brought on by high cortisol levels. This indicates that having a milkshake and french fries is more common than having a well-balanced dinner.

Reduced testosterone production is another effect of too much cortisol in the body. This might result in less muscle mass and a slower rate of calorie burning in the body. Since the metabolism is what turns food into energy, any alteration in this process could lead to a number of issues, including weight gain.

Moreover, persons who experience an increase in cortisol tend to gain weight around their abdomens. The term "toxic fat" refers to the fat that accumulates around the waist and is linked to the onset of cardiovascular disease.

Even while reducing stress may not always feel attainable on some days, increased cortisol can still have negative impacts that can be managed. This can be accomplished by engaging in relaxation techniques like deep breathing, yoga, meditation, or mindfulness to assist return this hormone's production to normal levels.

A diet rich in high-quality meals is necessary to avoid storing additional empty calories. Aim to consume a diet high in whole, plant-based meals, even when the body may be hankering after a fast fix. Naturally, choosing a healthy diet isn't always simple, but it's worthwhile. By keeping an eye on their diet, people may ensure that the calories they consume are transformed into energy rather than fat and stored by the body.

Lastly, one of the best ways to control stress hormones is through exercise. Exercise helps preserve lean body mass, whether a person chooses to work out at the gym, go for a run, or go for a regular stroll with family. This is particularly crucial when cortisol levels are elevated for extended periods of time.

CHAPTER 4 ~
STRATEGIES
FOR HORMONAL HARMONY

NUTRITION FOR HORMONAL BALANCE

Since specific nutrients are necessary for the synthesis, metabolism, and communication of hormones, nutrition is a critical factor in preserving hormonal equilibrium.

It's crucial to remember the following when attempting to enhance hormone health through diet:

1. Balanced Macronutrients: Eat a diet rich in appropriate proportions of healthy fats, carbs, and protein. Foods high in protein supply the critical amino acids needed for muscle repair and hormone synthesis.

Protein is essential for the synthesis of hormones, especially peptide hormones. These hormones, which are produced from amino acids, are essential for functions like energy metabolism and hunger control. Appropriate protein consumption aids in the synthesis of hormones that signal fullness and aid in appetite regulation, such as peptide YY (PYY) and glucagon-like peptide-1 (GLP-1).

Whole grains, fruits, and vegetables are good sources of complex carbs that help control blood sugar and avoid insulin spikes. Nutritious fats found in nuts, seeds, avocados, and fatty fish supply the vital fatty acids required for cellular activity and hormone production. Hormonal equilibrium is improved by including good fats in the diet. In addition to being required for the synthesis of several hormones, fats can aid in the treatment of insulin resistance, a condition in which cells fail to respond to insulin as intended, resulting in high blood sugar. Add foods high in omega-3 fatty acids, like walnuts, flaxseeds, chia seeds, and fatty fish (salmon, mackerel, and sardines). Omega-3 fatty acids promote hormone regulation, heart health, and brain function in addition to having anti-inflammatory qualities. Reduce your consumption of trans fats and harmful saturated fats, which are present in fried foods, processed foods, and fatty meats. Including fiber in your diet is crucial for enhancing the function of your hormones.

By managing gut health, which in turn can affect mental health, a diet rich in fiber from fruits, vegetables, and whole grains can enhance hormonal health. Fiber does not cause blood sugar increases since it does not convert to sugar.

2. Supportive Micronutrients: Make sure you're getting enough of the micronutrients that are necessary for hormone production, metabolism, and function. Important micronutrients are minerals like magnesium, zinc, and selenium, vitamins like D, B6, and E, and antioxidants like vitamin C and phytonutrients. These nutrients are essential for maintaining the functioning of the adrenal glands, thyroid, reproductive hormones, and insulin sensitivity.

3. Stabilize Blood Sugar: To avoid sharp spikes and crashes in blood sugar, concentrate on eating foods with a low glycemic index. These meals gradually release glucose into the bloodstream. Consume a diet high in fiber-rich foods, such as fruits, vegetables, legumes, whole grains, and slow-digesting meats, to help you feel fuller and more insulin-sensitive. Refined carbs, sweet meals,

and sugary drinks should be avoided in excess as they might upset blood sugar regulation and exacerbate insulin resistance.

4. Steer Clear of Endocrine Disruptors: Reduce your exposure to chemicals that cause endocrine disruption, such as those found in plastics, pesticides, household cleaners, and personal care items. Hormonal imbalances and detrimental consequences on health can result from EDCs interfering with hormone production, metabolism, and signalling. Whenever possible, choose natural, chemical-free personal care items, organic produce, and BPA-free plastics.

5. Control Alcohol and Caffeine: Restrict alcohol and caffeine intake as these substances can upset hormone balance and the stress response. While alcohol can obstruct liver detoxification and estrogen metabolism, caffeine can increase the release of cortisol and have an impact on adrenal function. It's important to exercise moderation, and making choices like herbal teas and mocktails can help maintain hormonal balance.

Because of its ability to promote hormonal health, eating a Mediterranean diet high in fruits, vegetables, lean proteins, and healthy fats is frequently advised. The focus of this diet plan is on foods that support general health and hormone balance.

6. Control Stress: Make use of stress-reduction strategies including yoga, deep breathing exercises, meditation, mindfulness, and getting enough sleep. Prolonged stress can throw off the balance of hormones by raising cortisol levels, which can cause abnormalities in thyroid, insulin, and reproductive hormones, among other hormones. To lessen the negative effects of stress on hormonal health, give relaxation, self-care, and good coping strategies first priority.

In summary, regular exercise and a well-balanced diet high in fiber, healthy fats, and protein can greatly support the maintenance of hormonal equilibrium. Your hormonal landscape is influenced by more than simply what you eat; it's also influenced by the way you live.

You may naturally balance your hormones by eating certain foods. The following is a list of foods with a reputation for balancing hormones:

Foods High in Protein: Including protein at every meal can affect hormones like peptide YY (PYY) and glucagon-like peptide-1 (GLP-1) that regulate hunger and food intake.

Fatty Fish: Foods high in omega-3 fatty acids, such as salmon, mackerel, and sardines, can help control hunger hormones.

Eggs: They positively affect the hormones ghrelin and insulin, which regulate hunger and blood sugar.

High-Fiber Carbohydrates: Complex carbohydrates with a high fiber content can lower cortisol levels and help stabilize blood sugar levels.

Good Fats: Including natural fats in your diet will help reduce insulin resistance and reduce hunger. Avocados, nuts, and seeds make excellent sources.

Cruciferous Vegetables: Broccoli and cauliflower are examples of vegetables that can support a normal hormonal balance.

Brazil nuts: Rich in selenium, which is necessary for the synthesis of thyroid hormones.

LIFESTYLE MODIFICATION TO SUPPORT HORMONAL HEALTH

A healthy endocrine system is maintained through lifestyle adjustments, which are crucial for sustaining hormonal health, an essential component of general well-being. Here are some lifestyle changes you may do to improve hormonal balance.

Sleep and Exposure to Light: Hormonal equilibrium depends critically on getting enough sleep. Sleep habits have an impact on the body's circadian rhythm, which controls hormones like melatonin and cortisol. Sleep disturbances can cause hormone imbalances, which in turn can exacerbate mood problems, stress, and weight gain. Aim for 7-9 hours of good sleep each night to support hormonal balance. Reduce your exposure to blue light from screens at night as well to avoid suppressing melatonin production, which can have an impact on hormone balance and the quality of your sleep.

Handling Stress: Extended periods of stress can significantly disrupt hormone levels, especially cortisol and adrenaline. When these stress hormones are increased for extended periods of time, they can interfere with other hormone activities. Stress management methods include deep breathing, mindfulness, and meditation. Stress reduction and hormone health are further benefits of indulging in joyful and relaxing hobbies.

Physical Activity: Hormonal health is significantly impacted by regular exercise. It lowers the chance of developing insulin resistance and aids in the regulation of hunger-controlling hormones like ghrelin and leptin. Increased endorphins from exercise can also elevate mood and lower stress levels. To support general hormonal balance, aim for a combination of cardiovascular, weight training, and flexibility workouts.

Dietary Decisions: Hormonal health is greatly influenced by diet. Eating a diet high in fiber, lean proteins, healthy fats, and whole foods can help to maintain the endocrine system. It is imperative to stay away from processed foods, high sugar content, and bad fats. Insulin resistance and other hormonal abnormalities may be exacerbated by them. Nutrients for hormone production and regulation can be obtained by including fatty fish, nuts, seeds, and legumes.

Chemical Exposure: Hormonal health depends on limiting exposure to endocrine disruptors, which are present in some plastics, cosmetics, and pesticides. To lessen your exposure to dangerous chemicals, choose natural and organic items wherever you can, and use glass or stainless steel containers rather than plastic ones.

Healthy Weight: Hormonal equilibrium depends on maintaining a healthy weight. Insulin resistance and the overproduction of some hormones, such estrogen, can result from excess fat, especially around the belly. A healthy weight can be attained and maintained with the help of a balanced diet and frequent exercise.

Hydration: In terms of hormonal health, adequate hydration is frequently disregarded. All biological processes, including the synthesis and movement of hormones, depend on water. For the sake of your general health and hormonal balance, try to consume at least 8 glasses of water each day.

Steer clear of Alcohol and Smoking: Both can have harmful impacts on the health of your hormones. They can cause a number of health problems and upset the hormone balance. Reducing alcohol use and giving up smoking can have a big impact on hormonal health.

Adopting these adjustments promotes general health and wellbeing in addition to the endocrine system. But one must always keep in mind that consistency is essential and that, over time, even modest adjustments can have a significant impact on hormonal health.

EXERCISE AND HORMONAL REGULATION

The control of hormones, which are essential for sustaining a number of biological processes like growth, metabolism, and mood, is greatly aided by exercise. The pancreas secretes the peptide hormone insulin, which controls how fat and carbohydrates are metabolized. Exercising improves the transport of nutrients and hormone signals, which helps lower insulin levels and increase insulin sensitivity. This helps control blood sugar levels.

Frequent exercise helps reduce the amounts of excess circulating estrogen, which is good for PMS symptoms and other conditions where estrogen is the dominating hormone.
Exercise also increases the release of endorphins, which are sometimes called "feel-good" hormones. These hormones have the potential to function as

natural painkillers in addition to enhancing mood and wellbeing.

The primary stress hormone in the body, cortisol, is influenced by physical exercise. While short-term increases in cortisol levels are possible with acute activity, regular exercise can help control cortisol production and lessen the damaging effects of long-term stress on the body.

Growth hormone, which is involved in the synthesis of muscle protein and tissue growth, can be released when exercising, particularly when high-intensity and resistance training is performed.

Ghrelin and leptin are the two hormones that control appetite. It has been demonstrated that exercise balances these hormones, which helps control satiety and hunger signals and aid in managing weight.

In conclusion, a variety of hormones that control different physiological responses in the body are influenced by exercise. It has the ability to be both catabolic, aiding in the breakdown of tissue, and anabolic, supporting the growth of new tissue. The hormones secreted and the effects they have on the body can be influenced by the kind and level of exercise. As a result, adding regular exercise to your lifestyle is a safe and efficient approach to promote hormonal balance and general health..

CHAPTER 5 ~ HORMONAL THERAPIES AND SUPPLEMENT

OVERVIEW OF HORMONAL REPLACEMENT THERAPY (HRT)

A medical procedure called hormone replacement therapy (HRT) is used to address symptoms of hormone shortages or imbalances, especially in menopausal women. The main objective of hormone replacement therapy (HRT) is to replenish the body's depleted levels of estrogen and progesterone. Menopause symptoms like vaginal dryness, hot flashes, and sweats can all be lessened with this. Oral tablets, transdermal patches, gels, lotions, and vaginal rings are just a few of the ways that hormone replacement therapy can be applied. The patient's symptoms, medical history, and preferences all play a role in the HRT selection process.

Better quality of life, increased bone density, and notable alleviation from menopausal symptoms are among the many advantages of hormone replacement therapy for many women. It might possibly have osteoporosis prevention benefits. Although HRT has the potential to provide relief, there are hazards involved. In certain people, they might include a higher risk of blood clots, stroke, breast cancer, and heart disease. After having a full discussion with your healthcare professional, taking into account your medical history and risk factors, you should decide whether to use HRT.

There is no one-size-fits-all approach to HRT. It should be customized to meet the needs of the patient, using the lowest effective dose for the shortest amount of time required to control symptoms. It is crucial to schedule routine check-ups with your healthcare practitioner in order to assess the efficacy of the therapy and make any necessary treatment adjustments.

HRT'S SIDE EFFECTS

Hormone Replacement Therapy (HRT) may cause a number of adverse effects, most of which go away with time. The following represent some side effects of HRT:

Estrogen Side Effects During HRT:

Headaches
tenderness or pain in the breasts
Unexpected spotting or bleeding in the vagina
emesis
Mood swings, such as despair or a bad mood
cramping in the legs
a little rash or irritation
The diarrhea
hair thinning

Progestogen Side Effects During HRT:

variations in the menstrual cycle, such as spotting or
intermenstrual bleeding
Headaches
tenderness or pain in the breasts
emesis
The diarrhea
Feeling worn out or lightheaded
Mood swings, such as despair or a bad mood
mild skin irritation or rash
Unknown

Some of the negative effects of progestogen or estrogen may manifest if you use combined hormone replacement therapy.

Tibolone Side Effects in HRT:

soreness in the breasts
Pelvic discomfort or stomach ache
unusual development of hair
Itching, vaginal discharge, or thrush
bleeding from the vagina.

In the first few months after beginning HRT, irregular vaginal bleeding or spotting is frequent; this usually goes away after six months. It's crucial to speak with your doctor if serious side effects arise or last longer than three months.

Keep in mind that not everyone will experience these possible side effects. It's also important to note that hormone replacement therapy (HRT) has advantages. Whether or not to take it depends on your own health history and risk factors, and should be decided after a careful consultation with your healthcare professional.

Menopausal symptoms can be managed with alternative medicines and lifestyle modifications for those who cannot or do not want to utilize HRT. These consist of non-hormonal medicines, frequent exercise, dietary changes, and stress-reduction strategies.

In conclusion, HRT is a helpful treatment for those who are having trouble adjusting to the consequences of hormonal changes, but it needs to be used carefully and tailored to the specific health needs of the patient.

NATURAL SUPPLEMENTS FOR HORMONAL BALANCE

Supplementing with natural vitamins can help maintain hormonal balance. Among the supplements that are frequently suggested are:

Magnesium: Involved in more than 300 enzymatic activities within the body, magnesium supports the endocrine system. It may lessen premenstrual symptoms, boost thyroid function, and assist control blood sugar levels.

Vitamin D: Often called the "sunshine vitamin," vitamin D is essential for immune system and bone health. It also affects how hormones like estrogen and testosterone are produced.

Growth hormone, insulin, and sex hormones are just a few of the hormones that need zinc to be produced and regulated. It can aid in the management of inflammation and is crucial for immune system function.

B vitamins: The metabolism and the synthesis of hormones and neurotransmitters depend on the B vitamins, especially B6, B12, and folate. They can promote adrenal health and aid with stress management.

Iodine: The production of thyroid hormones requires iodine. It has an impact on energy levels and metabolic rate. It should be used carefully though, as too much iodine can interfere with thyroid function.

Adaptogens: Because they assist the body in adjusting to stress, herbs such as ashwagandha and rhodiola rosea are referred to as adaptogens. They can promote general hormonal balance and control the release of stress hormones.

Probiotics: Hormonal health and gut health are related. A healthy gut microbiome is essential for hormone metabolism and detoxification, and probiotics can support this.

Omega-3 Fatty Acids: Found in flaxseeds and fish oil, omega-3 fatty acids boost the synthesis of hormones, including prostaglandins, which are anti-inflammatory and can help reduce inflammation.

CBD Oil: Due to its ability to alleviate stress, anxiety, and sleep disorders—all of which can impact hormonal balance—CBD oil is becoming more and more well-known. To completely comprehend its impact on hormones, more research is necessary, though.

It's crucial to remember that even while these supplements can help with hormonal health, a balanced diet and healthy lifestyle should always come first. Furthermore, as there may be interactions, it is imperative that you speak with your healthcare practitioner prior to beginning any new supplement regimen, particularly if you are taking medication or have a medical condition. Supplements ought to be used in conjunction with a healthy diet, regular exercise, stress reduction, and enough sleep as part of a holistic strategy for hormonal balance.

CHAPTER 6 ~ CASE STUDIES AND SUCCESS STORIES

REAL-LIFE EXAMPLES OF WOMEN ACHIEVING HORMONAL BALANCE AND WEIGHT MANAGEMENT GOALS

While I cannot provide personal stories without permission, I can share that many women have found success in achieving hormonal balance and weight management goals through a combination of diet, exercise, stress management, and sometimes medical interventions like Hormone Replacement Therapy (HRT). The women whose stories are mentioned below have their names changed to maintain anonymity.

Emma's Journey to Hormonal Harmony: Emma, a 35-year-old woman, struggled with polycystic ovary syndrome (PCOS), a hormonal disorder characterized by insulin resistance, irregular periods, and weight gain. After years of frustration with traditional diets and medications, Emma sought the guidance of a holistic healthcare provider who recommended a combination of dietary modifications, regular exercise, stress management techniques, and targeted supplements. By adopting a low-glycemic diet rich in whole foods, incorporating strength training and yoga into her fitness routine, practicing mindfulness and meditation, and taking supplements like inositol and omega-3 fatty acids, Emma was able to balance her hormones, regulate her menstrual cycle, improve insulin sensitivity, and achieve sustainable weight loss.

Sarah's Thyroid Transformation: Sarah, a 45-year-old woman, was diagnosed with hypothyroidism, a condition characterized by an underactive thyroid gland and symptoms such as fatigue, weight gain, and sluggish metabolism. Despite medication to support thyroid function, Sarah continued to struggle with weight management and felt discouraged by her slow progress. Determined to take control of her health, Sarah worked closely with a registered dietitian specializing in thyroid health and functional medicine. Together, they developed a personalized nutrition plan focused on supporting thyroid function, balancing blood sugar levels, and optimizing nutrient intake. By incorporating thyroid-supportive foods like seaweed, brazil nuts, and bone broth, minimizing inflammatory foods like gluten and processed sugars, and prioritizing stress management and adequate sleep, Sarah's energy levels, metabolism, and weight loss all significantly improved.

Jessica's Journey to Overcome Menopausal Challenges: Jessica, a 55-year-old woman, faced hormonal changes associated with menopause, including fluctuations in estrogen and progesterone levels, hot flashes, and abdominal weight gain. Frustrated by her inability to lose weight despite strict dieting and exercise, Jessica sought the expertise of a menopause specialist and certified personal trainer. Together, they developed a comprehensive approach to address Jessica's hormonal imbalances and weight management goals. By incorporating hormone-balancing foods like cruciferous vegetables, flaxseeds, and soy products into her diet, engaging in strength training and high-intensity interval training (HIIT) workouts to boost metabolism and muscle mass, and prioritizing self-care practices such as acupuncture and massage therapy to alleviate menopausal symptoms, Jessica was able to achieve hormonal balance, improve body composition, and enhance her overall quality of life.

These real-life examples demonstrate that achieving hormonal balance and weight management goals often requires a personalized and holistic approach that addresses underlying imbalances, supports metabolic health, and promotes sustainable lifestyle changes. By working with knowledgeable healthcare professionals and adopting evidence-based strategies tailored to individual needs, women can overcome hormonal challenges and achieve long-term success in their health and wellness journey. Keep in mind that every person's journey is different, so what suits one person might not suit another.

CHAPTER 7 ~ *CONCLUSION*

RECAP OF KEY CONCEPTS

I appreciate you joining me on this adventure. The main ideas discussed in the book "Beyond Weight Loss for Women: The Role and Effect of Hormones in Weight Loss" are summarized here.

1. Realizing Hormonal Complexity: Losing weight involves a complicated interaction of hormonal variables and is not only about balancing calories in and out. Hormones that control metabolism, hunger, fat storage, and energy balance include estrogen, progesterone, insulin, cortisol, and thyroid hormones.

2. Effect of Hormonal Imbalance: Hormone imbalances can interfere with metabolic processes, cause weight gain or trouble shedding weight, and have an adverse effect on general health and well-being. They can also result from stress, nutrition, lifestyle choices, medical problems, or genetic predispositions.

3. Holistic Weight Management: Using a holistic weight management strategy entails treating hormonal imbalances in their entirety through dietary changes, lifestyle adjustments, stress reduction methods, physical activity, and, if required, pharmacological interventions.

4. Nutritional Techniques for Hormonal Balance: Maintaining hormonal balance is greatly aided by nutrition. Consuming a diet rich in balanced macronutrients, emphasizing micronutrients that assist blood sugar regulation, controlling stress, avoiding endocrine disruptors, controlling alcohol and caffeine intake, and stabilizing blood sugar levels are all important dietary strategies.

5. Lifestyle Modifications: Hormonal balance and the results of weight control can be significantly impacted by lifestyle factors like physical exercise, sleep hygiene, stress management, and environmental exposures. Making healthy lifestyle adjustments can help support long-term weight loss and hormonal balance.

6. Personalized Interventions: Since every woman's hormonal profile and weight reduction journey are different, it is crucial to provide individualized care that meets her requirements and preferences in order to get the best outcomes. Seeking advice from medical specialists, such as functional medicine practitioners, endocrinologists, or registered dietitians, can offer tailored direction and assistance.

7. Empowerment and Long-Term Success: Women can empower themselves to achieve hormonal balance, optimize metabolic health, and reach sustainable weight management goals by comprehending the complexities of hormone regulation, implementing evidence-based strategies, and actively participating in their health and wellness journey.

All things considered, "Beyond Weight Loss for Women: The Role and Effect of Hormones in Weight Loss" offers a thorough grasp of the complex interplay between hormones and weight control, giving women the information and resources they need to manage their hormonal health and succeed long-term in their weight loss efforts.

EMPOWERING WOMEN TO TAKE CONTROL OF THEIR HORMONAL HEALTH AND WEIGHT LOSS JOURNEY

To feel empowered, women must take charge of their health. Encouraging women to take charge of their weight management and hormonal health requires a complex strategy that includes support, education, and resource access.

Education: The key to power is knowledge. The first step is to comprehend how hormones impact the body, emotions, and metabolism. Comprehensive information on the science of hormones and how they affect women's health may be found at sites like FEMM Health. It is essential to understand the functions of various hormones and how lifestyle choices can affect them.

Personalized Health Tracking: Women's tracking of their menstrual cycles and symptoms can yield important information on the state of their hormones. Women can learn to spot patterns and any anomalies that may require medical care by using journals or apps.

Nutrition and Diet: It's critical to inform women about the value of a balanced diet that promotes hormonal equilibrium. Consuming complete foods and healthy fats is part of this, as avoiding processed meals and high sugar intake can result in hormone imbalances.

Physical Activity: Exercising on a regular basis helps balance hormones and regulate weight. It can raise hormones that elevate mood, lower stress hormones, and increase insulin sensitivity.

Stress Reduction: Hormonal equilibrium can be upset by prolonged stress. Stress management methods include deep breathing, yoga, and meditation. Counseling and support groups can also be sources of emotional well-being and stress reduction.

Medical Support: It's critical to have access to medical specialists who are knowledgeable on hormone health. Whether it's through hormone replacement therapy (HRT) or other therapies, women should feel at ease sharing their worries and symptoms with their doctors and getting the care they need.

Community and Support: It can be immensely empowering for women to be able to share their experiences, struggles, and victories in a community setting. Women might be inspired and motivated to take control of their health by their peers' support.

Supplements and Alternative Therapies: Natural supplements and alternative therapies may provide relief for certain ladies. It's crucial to speak with medical professionals before beginning any new supplementation or treatment, though.

Having knowledge to make decisions regarding one's health leads to empowerment. Women can take charge of their weight loss and hormonal health by giving them the resources, information, and encouragement they require. This will enhance their well-being and quality of life. Keep in mind that each woman has a unique figure, so what suits one might not suit another. It's about figuring out what works best for each person and striking the correct balance.

CHAPTER 8 ~ RESOURCES
AND FURTHER READING

Here are some resources that can provide additional information on hormonal health and weight management for your further reading:

Books:

"WomanCode" by Alisa Vitti

"TheHormoneCure"byDr. SaraGottfried

"Period Repair Manual" and "Hashimoto's Food Pharmacology" are also highly regarded in the field of endocrinology

---

Websites:

Cleveland Clinic offers comprehensive information on hormonal imbalances and treatments.

The Hormone Health Network provides trusted information to understand hormone-related conditions and treatment options.

MedlinePlus is a valuable resource for information on hormones and endocrine glands.

Professionals:

Endocrinologists specialize in metabolism and hormonal changes and can help with weight management related to hormone conditions.

The North American Menopause Society has a directory to find menopause practitioners.

For personalized care, platforms like Zocdoc can help locate female hormone specialists near you.

These resources can be a great starting point for anyone looking to deepen their understanding of hormonal health and weight management. Remember to consult with healthcare professionals before making any significant changes to your health regimen.

REVIEW REQUEST

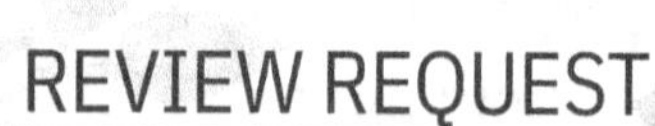

Dear Reader,

I hope this message finds you well. I am reaching out to request your valuable feedback on my latest book, "Beyond Weight Loss; The Role and Effects of Hormones on Weight Loss"

I believe your insights would be incredibly valuable in evaluating the content, accuracy, and overall impact of the book. "Beyond Weight Loss; The Role and Effects of Hormones on Weight Loss" delves into the complex relationship between hormones and weight management, offering practical strategies, evidence-based insights, and personalized interventions tailored specifically for women's health.

Your honest review would not only provide valuable feedback for me as an author but also help prospective readers make informed decisions about whether the book aligns with their needs and goals. Your opinion matters greatly, and I would be deeply grateful for your time and consideration in sharing your thoughts.

Thank you in advance for considering my request. Your support means the world to me, and I look forward to hearing from you soon.

Warm regards,

Mosier, Ann R.